"I HAVE SEEN YOUR TEARS"

Notes of Support
From a Fellow Sufferer

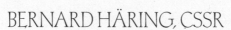

BERNARD HÄRING, CSSR

TRANSLATED BY
Robert Hodge, OCSO

LIGUORI
PUBLICATIONS
One Liguori Drive
Liguori, MO 63057-9999
314-464-2500

Originally published as „Ich habe deine Trähen gesehan" © Verlag Herder Freiburg im Breisgau 1993.

Scriptural citations are taken from the *New Revised Standard Version of the Bible,* copyright © 1989 by the Division of Christian Education of the National Council of the Churches of Christ in the USA. All rights reserved. Used with permission.

Cover design by Myra Roth

I have heard your prayer,
I have seen your tears,
indeed, I will heal you…

2 Kings 20:5

ABOUT THE AUTHOR

Redemptorist Bernard Häring, CSSR, is a renowned moral theologian and author of over eighty books. His major works include the multi-volume sets *The Law of Christ* (1954) and *Free and Faithful in Christ* (1978, 1980).

He was born on November 10, 1912, the son of devout German parents, and the eleventh of twelve children. His eventful life has covered apocalyptic times. His childhood saw the ravages of World War I, and his coming of age coincided with the rise of Hitler and National Socialism.

As a young priest, he was drafted into the Wehrmacht medical corps. He served the military and civilian populations of France, Poland, and Russia in both a medical and religious capacity. During the German retreat from Stalingrad, Father Häring convinced his fellow soldiers to throw down their guns and to follow him to safety; he himself was saved from a Russian prisoner-of-war camp through the help of an entire Polish parish.

After the war, he returned to Germany where he completed his doctoral studies in 1947, and became a teacher of moral theology at Gars am Inn. During this time he also ministered to the refugees of Europe as an itinerant pastor.

Father Häring was then assigned to teach moral theology in Rome and participated in the preparatory work of the Second Vatican Council, as well as its official proceedings.

In the 1970s and early 1980s, Father Häring faced not only a painful examination of his work by the Congregation for the Doctrine of the Faith, but also a long and death-defying battle with cancer of the throat. As a result of this illness, Father Häring lost his voice and had to learn to speak anew.

Father Häring—after distinguished worldwide contributions—now lives in Germany.

CONTENTS

INTRODUCTION

Certainly there is no individual or family that has not had to deal with sorrow and sickness— some more, others less. This dialogue with sorrow and sickness goes with our being human.

The real questions arising as a result of this dialogue are, above all, these: Will it be of any use to hold a dialogue with sickness? What purpose is served by our faith when sorrow and sickness strike? What are the powers that flow into us from our faith when it arises out of these circumstances?

At times we experience faith as a bodily healing power. But this kind of healing, though not impossible, is less likely or less frequent. If, on the other hand, we look to faith to give meaning to our suffering, then healing is much more likely to take place and to occur more frequently.

It is not my intent here to launch a theological discussion about the value of illness as faith-enhancing but to follow the story-telling approach—to join the fellowship of people who have come to terms with illness even though it has struck them down with a heavy hand. I wish to boldly tell the story of my own acquaintance with illness, not to portray myself as an example, but to narrate a story in which even widely different readers will recognize themselves.

I would not have decided to write my story if it were not for the fact that I have been asked, on the strength of my own experiences with sickness and sorrow, to write some kind of book of consolation for sick people and to stretch out a helping hand to those who look after them. I cannot imagine a greater joy than knowing that those who are suffering gain comfort and strength through the sharing of our faith experiences.

— *Bernard Häring*
Gars, Germany

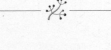

PART I

The Lessons
of
Sickness and Suffering

—— ✼ ——

LESSONS FROM
THE SICKNESS OF OTHERS

We are not attacked by sickness completely alone. We experience it within the skein of family, friends, and those who have something to say to us. I learned of the shocking facts of sickness and sorrow as a healthy six-year-old among a healthy brood of brothers and sisters.

Toward the end of World War I, my mother experienced a life-threatening hemorrhage. We children all depended on her, no less than did our father, for whom she was the living gospel.

How anxious we all were about our mother's very life. We all prayed, and we children behaved in an exemplary fashion in order to spare our parents any deeper trouble than they already had.

Soon after my mother fell ill, the postman arrived with two letters. Obviously to him, the letters brought the news that my two elder brothers, who were stationed at the Front, were counted among the missing. Being a man of sensitive feelings, the postman brought the letters to a woman relative of ours who delivered the news to us.

We all broke into tears, and our father told us to be sure not to enter our sick mother's room with tears in our eyes, or "else mother will die as well." Believing that any tears in their eyes were no longer visible, my two elder sisters visited our mother's sick room. At once she noticed their uneasiness and asked, "Which of the two is fallen?"

My mother survived her illness and later it turned out that only my eldest brother had fallen. The second eldest brother came home a year later from imprisonment in England sick with a rare form of cancer of the neck.

His illness hit my father with particular severity, since my brother Wenzel had joined the army voluntarily in order to save our father from conscription into war service. Father had forbidden him to volunteer, but Wenzel stood his ground and bravely took our father's place.

Father did all he could to find the best doctor to treat Wenzel's illness. [Editor's note: In Bernard Häring's *My Witness for the Church* (Mahwah, NJ: Paulist Press, 1992) Wenzel's illness is identified as lupus which he had contracted while a prisoner.] In the end, a professor of medicine in Tubingen was able to help by urging my brother to take up the fight against this illness with the weapon of vegetarianism. So, my brother waged a war against his illness that included both the healing power of prayer and the beneficial effects of a meatless diet. ✳

PRAYERFUL HEALINGS

Two other instances of the illuminating power of prayer were of special significance to me when I came to face my own illnesses. In my youth, my family took care of an elderly woman named Cecilia who was blind and quite poor because of Germany's raging rate of inflation.

I often had the honor of bringing warm food or a loaf of bread to her. From an initial feeling of sympathy, there grew up in me a deep respect for this good and utterly God-dedicated woman. Through her, this fact was impressed on my memory: one can radiate joy even though sick, elderly, and poor.

Then, as a young priest, I was a guest preacher for a week in a parish in Lower Bavaria where even the young people and children—as well as their parents—were keenly attentive to my preaching. This in itself was edifying, but also in evidence was the faith manifested by many parishioners in the way they sought the will of God in their daily life.

Remarking on this, I said to the parish priest: "Nowhere have I found such faith. Could you let me in on the secret of your parishioners' concern for spirituality?"

His answer was this: "The secret lies neither with me

nor with my curate. If you wish to get behind the secret, then visit a sick woman of our parish who has been bedridden for decades. Now she is so badly afflicted that she cannot even raise her hand to her mouth."

I visited her poor apartment where I found a woman not racked with pain but radiating bliss. Her face was not distorted with suffering, but rather her eyes were beaming light and goodness.

I remember her words: "Father, I cannot thank God enough that my sickness and my sorrows are redeemed, and I can cooperate in the work of redemption." She was speaking not of needful expiation for the sins of others, but quite simply of redemption as a gift received and as a present to be passed on.

The parish priest told me after my visit: "It seems to me that this sick woman has become the center for the proclamation of the Good News for our parish, a proclamation made without the wordiness of our preaching." ✼

FACING MY ILLNESSES

I am writing now as a man of eighty years presently in outstanding health and full of the joy of life. Yet because of the story of the bleak periods of my illnesses, the thought might occur to some readers that I am almost a man of suffering like Job.

This similarity is not strictly true for two reasons. In the first place, the question "Why?" never bothered me as it did the man of suffering in Old Testament days. And, secondly, before me always stood the figure of the crucified and risen Lord—a sight not granted to Job. Because of this vision, I knew that I was approaching near to the key of understanding and acceptance. Nevertheless, I must state that despite these differences, I wrestled with questions similar to those that faced Job. ✣

NATURE HEALS

I entered the Redemptorist novitiate in Deggendorf in 1933 in the peak of youth and health. I was athletic and held my own in gymnastics. Very soon, I discovered that my respected novice master took great exception to my gymnastic exercises in the cloister garden. Then and there, I gave them up.

As well, under the instruction of this same novice master, I also gave up kneeling down—a choice that resulted in great bodily stress and tension. Additionally, I took up a physical practice prescribed by him to attain an abiding awareness of the Presence of God. With great pains and determination, I followed his prescriptions, determined to repel every distraction.

The result was soon apparent: "Stretched too taut, the bow snaps." Almost at once, heaviness of heart and persistent headaches set in.

Meanwhile the novitiate was transferred to Gars where the local doctor was bound to the monastery by friendly ties. Seeing that healthwise I could not cope, he urged me to abandon the idea of a religious vocation once and for all.

He also passed on this conclusion to the novice master and warned him strongly: "This young man will only be a burden to the monastery. He will never again arrive at a full working capacity."

The novice master, who was devoted to me, was in tears as he told me of the doctor's conclusion. For confirmation, he took me to a famous eye specialist. She not only gave me a basic eye examination, but she used every means available at that time for a broader diagnosis.

Her results were passed on to the novice master as well: "Keep this young man calm. But give him more opportunity for recreation and relaxation. He should also take up gymnastics again, only step by step, of course."

The monastery decided to take a risk with me. When I took my vows in May, 1934, I was on the road to recovery, although kneeling in front of the altar was still beyond me. I took my vows seated on a chair. What a risk on both sides!

My immediate superior in the scholasticate at Rothenfeld, Father Engelbert Zettl, teacher of church history, was a man of wisdom and goodness who allowed me every freedom for my convalescence.

He lectured during the third period every day. And, although church history was of great interest to me, I generally fell asleep for some ten minutes during his class.

When I asked him one day if he had noticed that I often fell asleep during his lecture and what did he think of it, his answer took me by surprise yet showed his natural empathy: "What ought I to think? Hopefully, the sleep did you good!" Yes, indeed! It is these kinds of human relationships that do good as well!

In addition to the kindness of Father Zettl, I also encountered the healing effects of the world of nature. Soon after my entry into the scholasticate, a small roebuck was injured and a second one was caught in a trap.

I took a strong liking to these two little creatures, feeding them at first from a milk bottle. Not only did they trustfully feed from my hand, they also provided me with racing competition.

The chance to get out of the trap of preoccupation with my own health meant more for my healing than any order to "relax." Nothing is worse for the sick than continual absorption and care about one's own health. Orders for relaxation and diversion can be highly overrated if not executed in terms of some real meaningful activity taken up for itself and not for the sake of the illness.

From 1935 until the time of my being seriously wounded in battle in May of 1942, I never again needed to see a doctor. ✳

THE SICKNESS OF WAR

S oon after the beginning of World War II in
1939, I was drafted into the medical corps of
the German army and sent to Munich and
Augsburg for training. From January to September
of 1940, I was given a leave of absence to teach moral
theology.

Then I was transferred to an infantry regiment in
France where I had the duty of looking after the health
of my comrades. This duty gave me an important
pastoral contact, while providing me also with a certain
amount of embarrassment, since my duties included
the prevention of sexual diseases and the medical care
of soldiers after sexual intercourse with prostitutes.

I was also made responsible for the health service of
a brothel provided for soldiers, and it rested with me
to appoint the first-aid workers for the routine health
service there.

Briefly, I can only say that in these marginal situations we were able to forestall a great deal of evil and
promote a great deal of good. It was possible, for
example, for many a young girl to be set free from
prostitution, and for many a man to be persuaded to
do some serious thinking.

Delicate tasks of a similar nature were to trouble me again during the Russian campaign—my next duty assignment. There I had to give notice of cases of sexual infection and to isolate their sources in order to prevent further outbreaks.

When a young journalist from our battalion caught an infection from a married woman, mother of several children, and the situation made it impossible to send the woman away for treatment, my harsh regimental commander ordered me to have the woman shot.

I could have made it clear to my commander that he certainly could not expect anything of the kind from a priest, but in that case, someone else would have been given the order and carried it out.

So I accepted the responsibility and told the woman that now my own life lay in her hands should she pass the infection on to anyone else again. I trusted her assurance—as was right—never again to give the infection to anyone and to take the prescribed medicine regularly. This incident shows again how life and health are entrusted to all of us collectively.

During the war, sickness, sorrow, and death arose in an entirely new way with the most unheard of sharpness. In the first hour of the Russian war, a bomb splinter struck a Jesuit friend standing beside me and shattered his brain. As his whole body reared up mightily, I uttered a bitter "Why?" And then, one hour later, I was taking care of the first seriously wounded soldiers.

What we medical orderlies were able to do was much; yet in light of the amount of death and suffering as a whole, we could accomplish almost nothing.

From this war experience emerged in me the vocation to work for the cause of peace and the healing power of nonviolence. This is the work that I still had to do by way of my own suffering for "by his bruises we are healed" (Isaiah 53:5).

May all who call themselves Christians work hard for the healing power of freedom, for redemptive dedication to the abolition of hostility with an eye on the Slave of God, Jesus Christ, so as to bring salvation and healing to the whole of humanity.

This is my answer to the vexatious "Why?" No one should stand still in the face of the "Why?", but instead should enroll themselves among the apostles for the healing power of nonviolence as the way to peace. ✵

LIVING WITH BROTHER DEATH

As a medical sergeant major in an infantry regiment, I lived with death as enemy number one. This is so even though I happened to have the experience of redemption through contact with believers who hand themselves over to Brother Death with an eye on the One who has risen from the dead.

In one such experience, I hurried to bring help to a wounded soldier belonging to an evangelical denomination. As I was undoing his clothing, his intestines gushed out.

Acting as a priest I said to him: "Say *yes*; the Father is calling you home." The soldier answered: "If God is calling me, I am always ready." These words meant more to me than a whole treatise about sickness, sorrow, and death.

In a senseless and cruel war, it is difficult to follow the path of Saint Francis of Assisi and make friends with death as a brother. Yet I attempted to do this—for a redeeming death in the service of the wounded was a means of escape from the horrific vale of tears in which I found myself. Throughout the entire war, even during a break in Stuttgart and a heavy bomb attack,

I tried to get on friendly terms with the possible closeness of Brother Death.

In May of 1942, during a big battle at a location between Kharkov and Kursk, Brother Death appeared to be quite near. I had lost all five of the stretcher bearers in my infantry battalion when a splinter from a hand grenade injured me in the head. The splinter penetrated like fire and in a few minutes my clothes were all bloody.

With my last ounce of strength, I bandaged myself enough to prevent my bleeding to death. I can still remember the scene when someone handed me into a large first-aid station, and the Russian helper who had to remove my blood-soaked clothing began to weep loudly.

His weeping unnerved me, since the first and last time I had wept during the war was when, at the beginning, I gave my Jesuit friend the anointing of the sick at his last gasp. It was clear to me, that if I was to go any further in my expression of compassion, my spiritual collapse would soon follow. It simply meant that on all occasions of sympathy, I must again and again bite my tongue and master myself.

My comrades often expressed amazement at how calmly I gave my assistance even in the most difficult of cases. They had no inkling how my blood-stained hands, the sight and the wounds of the wounded, disturbed me in my dreams. These nightmares continued for years after the war whenever the strain on my nerves was too severe.

There have been further opportunities after the war to support men as they lay dying—men who have gone home so utterly at peace with themselves and with God that I could be healed of serious soul-wounds inflicted by the oft-repeated experience of violent death in the war.

In this respect I am thinking above all of my Roman colleague, Father Dressino, in whom I always saw the ideal priest and colleague. As he had an inkling that death was close at hand, he expressed the wish that I should give him the anointing of the sick. What peace I saw on his face!

A couple of hours after receiving the sacrament for the sick, he turned to me and asked, "What is the name of the priest who wrote that fine book *Yes, Father*?" When I answered: "Richard Graf," he said in a low voice but quite understandably, "Now I am saying this prayer for the last time: 'Yes, Father!'"

Then early in the morning when the nurse found him and asked him how he was, he replied, "I am blissfully happy!" These were his last words.

MISDIAGNOSIS AND ITS AFTERMATH

In the second winter of the war in Russia, typhus appeared in our unit. As a sergeant in the medical corps, I had correctly diagnosed more than a few cases of this disease among soldiers as well as civilians, and was also—to some extent—able to give the right kind of help.

Our newly appointed medical practitioner brought a sick man to me whom, he hoped, I would nurse back to health in a short time. I warned the doctor: "This man has typhus. We must take him at once to a casualty clearing station; tomorrow he will no longer be movable."

The otherwise sympathetic doctor felt he was not being respected as a doctor and refused to acknowledge my diagnosis of typhus. Only after some days did he allow me to bring him to the field dispensary, where I told the doctor in charge that, in my opinion, this man had a case of abdominal typhus.

The doctor ordered me to stay at the field dispensary until my own diagnosis had been verified. For if I had slept over a period of three days anywhere near this man, I was a candidate for the sick bay as well. Nevertheless, I went back to my post where I was badly needed.

Typhus doesn't keep you waiting long. I was felled by the illness. I quarantined myself in the assembly room, not allowing anyone near me. It was too late for me to return to the clearing station. It was not only the virus which I had to battle, but also the vexation of the wrong diagnosis—a typical eventuality with which many of the sick must deal.

Eventually the doctor involved in this case himself had to go to the hospital with spotted fever. At that point, the colonel insisted that I should be responsible for the whole of the medical service, since he did not have much confidence in the young doctors currently being sent to the front after completing only the barest minimum of scientific formation.

Thus, for nearly a year, I carried the responsibility for the entire medical operation for my group. I found this spiritually almost unbearable, until I decided to go straight to the head of the medical corps and lay before him my concerns. After this appeal, we got an excellent physician, and once again I could breathe.

THE HEALING POWER
OF COMPOSURE

After my return to civilian life, I was still suffering from the effects of the illnesses and privations brought on by the war—the aftermath of typhus and the effects of jaundice, thoroughly treated, but not at the right time.

All this scarcely affected my joy in life and my creative energy. One of the reasons, indeed the basic reason, was my delight in my vocation from which I gained a rich harvest of love and gratitude.

The year 1954 saw the publication of my three-volume work on moral theology entitled *The Law of Christ.* Reactions to this publication, however, were a heavy burden to me and resulted in psychosomatic consequences.

Possibly because of my growing influence on the renewal of moral theology, some groups of the theological rearguard took me to task through the Holy Office. Their complaints mainly focused on the questions of situation ethics and the burial of obedience to the law.

Weekly letters of complaints against me were sent to

the Superior General of my Order; and also these same kinds of letters were sent to the Holy Office. From that time on, the orthodoxy of my three-volume work of moral theology *The Law of Christ* was examined by the Holy Office under a magnifying glass. Even so, I participated in the work of the preparatory commission for the Second Vatican Council by arrangement of Pope John XXIII.

At this time I experienced serious abdominal pains, and I embarked on a thorough medical examination which uncovered an intestinal ulcer almost thirty centimeters long. The anxious attending doctor encouraged me to withdraw from all stressful and burdensome duties, and above all, from my work in Rome.

After listening to him for thirty minutes, I said: "Dear doctor, I am not going to abandon my responsibilities to the Church. But, from today on, I shall pray for composure and drill myself in its practice."

Others joined with me in my intention; and, in my opinion, our prayers were heard. I recovered without extensive use of medication and without following an ultra-strict diet. I credit composure as a great source of healing power; but this power—after all—is a gift of God. ✺

WORK NOURISHES HEALTH

T he Second Vatican Council demanded of me quite a large measure of work—work of such a kind that through it a person is able to see his or her own proper responsibility and limits. Because of my work on the theological commission of the Council, I had innumerable discussions with Council fathers and Council theologians, and also with observers from other Christian churches at the Council. Added to that were numerous lectures in different languages for larger groups of bishops.

For me, the Second Vatican Council was an absolute spiritual high. My creative energy seemed almost limitless, and physically I seemed indefatigable. But, by the end of the Council and very soon after, it soon appeared to me that I had expected too much and had overestimated the situation of the Church.

In the midst of my disillusionment, a heart specialist diagnosed a very severe heart condition and prescribed a very strong remedy. When I asked him how long I had to go on taking these medications, he answered laconically, "Always." To my question, "What does that mean?" he answered, "Until your blissful end."

Even with the added burden of a seemingly permanent heart condition, I remained joyfully active and determined to see my part of the work of the Council to the very end. I refused to put the brakes on any of my work-related activities.

Amazingly, after eighteen months, a distinguished medical adviser, who trusted my judgment of my own health, advised me to gradually get rid of all of my medications. This solution succeeded beyond my highest expectations.

Without a strain on my health even worth mentioning, I could continue my sabbatical from my academic work and serve in the mission and spread of the work of the Council, especially in Africa, Asia, and America.

During this time, I often needed a day of fasting, yet I never needed special food. I nourished myself, so to speak, on my joy in the service of the Gospel and on the unspoken love that streamed all over me.

My own experiences—as well as scientific study—have convinced me that the most decisive health factor is the quality of human relationships. In the same vein, however, mental and physical composure are also factors that should not be overlooked.

CANCER AND DENIAL

In June of 1975 the scrutiny of my work by the Vatican culminated in a formal teaching investigation by the Holy Office. Even though this examination affected the excellence of my health, it did not reduce my joy in working in the service of the Gospel and the cause of ecumenism over the next several years.

On the feast of Corpus Christi in 1977 I was presiding at High Mass in the church of Fordham University in New York City. Suddenly, to my surprise, all the higher notes were beyond my vocal reach. Never in all my years as a priest had I suffered from hoarseness, since I had an excellent voice and exceptionally good voice training. In a very short time, my voice faded to a whisper.

I could have known what was wrong, but at the same time, I wished not to know it. This unexpected hoarseness was a symptom of cancer of the throat. This refusal to acknowledge what was happening was the way it was with many a cancer victim and still is. One simply refuses to believe it, although at bottom of it, one is aware that the cancer is there.

The first sign of cancer came almost simultaneously

with the verdict from Rome as a result of its teaching investigation. This verdict brought even greater difficulties for me to bear, and created an even greater constellation of unfavorable factors that had a psycho-somatic bearing on my health. ❧

GRATITUDE AS A HEALER

While still in New York at Fordham University, I took a walk one afternoon through the Bronx. Arriving back home, I discovered that I had lost my keys. Before darkness fell, I determined to retrace my steps, hoping vainly to find the bunch of keys. After an unsuccessful search, I returned to the Jesuit house where I was living, where the Superior assured me that he would provide me with a fresh set of keys on the following day.

That night I had a dream. In this dream, I saw my bunch of keys lying on the ledge of a street pillar. In this dream, I thanked God with all my heart that he had shown me the keys.

I awoke refreshed at the break of day, and went into the city. I went up to a pillar on a wide street and there, in reality, lay my bunch of keys. Rubbing my eyes, I reassured myself that it wasn't a dream but the fullness of reality. Only shortly before, I had read something written by a man whom I held in great honor, Mahatma Gandhi. To paraphrase, he said, prayer as an expression of trust and gratitude is the key both for the evening and for the morning; in the morning especially, it opens our life to the light.

Now I knew in a flash that I had found not only the keys to the house of the Jesuits, to my room and to my office, but also I had found the key to mastering my current situation—the Vatican teaching investigation plus the throat cancer.

I was firmly convinced that God in his fatherly care had given the key into my hand. I was bursting with trust and made a firm resolution to learn more solidly what was meant by "always and on every occasion to be thankful; that is the way of salvation and healing."

Certainly my self-deception, so typical of cancer victims, was not yet fully overcome. My doctor had assured me that my hoarseness was only a matter of polyps, although I knew perfectly well that ear-nose-and-throat doctors are in the habit of saying that. I wanted to cling to these threads of hope that, with the removal of the polyps, all would be clear.

The operation took place in the clinic of the Grey Sisters in Rome, which was situated adjacently to where I was staying. After the preliminary operation, as I gazed at the faces of the doctor and attending sister who were good friends of mine, I knew at once what was the matter. My self-deception was over; the search phase had begun. ✣

THE FULLNESS OF
GOD'S HELP

As I began my search for the next steps, I talked over my situation with Professor Fratarcangelo who said: "You may be in luck. I learned a method in the United States of renewing cancerous vocal cords by means of new ones taken from the patient's own mucous membranes. It is, of course, taken for granted that the patient is not a smoker, for mucous membranes affected by tobacco smoke are not suitable.

He also gave me to understand that the hospital situated south of Rome in Colleferro, where he was able to operate as senior surgeon, was poorly furnished even though it did not lack the basics.

I made up my mind to entrust myself to this very capable and humanly sympathetic doctor. To my superior he said, "If God helps us, Father Häring will recover somewhere in the range of fifty percent of the volume of his former voice."

To everyone's astonishment, it turned out that I got back almost the full strength, and the full ring of my previous voice—a masterly achievement of the doctors who operated on me and took care of me. ✄

CORDIALITY SOFTENS AFFLICTION

The ward of the hospital where those suffering from throat diseases were assigned could accommodate up to twenty-five patients. But for this entire group, only one single and unbelievably primitive toilet was available. Even so, good spirits among the patients and staff prevailed.

Very shortly after my arrival, members of a charismatic renewal group from the Colleferro district came to greet me. They brought me a handsome flowering plant as well as a knife, fork, and spoon. They had suspected that I did not know that the patients had to bring these utensils themselves.

Every day, one member of this prayer group came to see if I was in need of any kind of attention. Their self-giving, self-understanding, and sincerity of heart did me good.

Near me in the ward was an eighty-year-old impoverished noblewoman who was also a patient. She came to visit me with an amiable laugh and encouraged me with the words, "I am stone deaf, and you are quite dumb; in the end, it comes to the same thing."

Her tone of voice and her laugh made music. And as she noticed how her sympathy visits improved my mood, she came to visit more often, and with her fine voice, sang me a song.

From all sides came fountains of cordiality to which I responded, not indeed with words but with a good laugh. I never had any regrets for having decided in favor of this hospital intended for the poor, not only because my doctor fulfilled all my highest expectations but also because of the experience of the most cordial human relationships in the midst of affliction.

GRATITUDE DRIVES
OUT FEAR

Just prior to the operation on my throat, which was expected to take five hours, a young nun who was also a nurse came to administer the pre-operation injections. She looked at me in astonishment, and said, "How can you, before so serious an operation, look so happy?"

As I was not able to speak, I answered her on my little tablet which could be immediately wiped clean: "That is pure grace. And, if I were not being continually grateful, such happiness would be immediately lost."

Still, because of my enforced silence, I could not tell her fully where this happy feeling came from. Before she arrived, I had had a deep, restful sleep during which the following dream occurred: In a wonderful valley I saw Jesus, the Good Shepherd. He nodded to me as though he would invite me to follow him. I was full of joy.

After waking up, I interpreted the dream in this manner: So, now, you may leave this vale of tears. Yes, Jesus himself has invited me.

Then sleep overtook me again, and I had a totally different dream: I was running all the way to the railway ticket office to buy the "big" ticket. But whenever I looked, there was someone nodding politely. Thus, my interpretation of these dreams had to be revised. I concluded that the time for the final journey had not yet come, but the invitation of the Good Shepherd remains. ⚘

SUCCESSFUL SURGERY UNDER HYPNOSIS

The condition of my blood and the state of my liver were other than good. This coupled with the length of the operation resulted in my doctor's choosing hypnosis as an anesthesia rather than the more traditional means.

My doctor had not gone into much detail about anesthesia by hypnosis, so I had no idea of what to expect when I finally arrived in the operating room. There I was given an injection, and the anesthetist talked to me intently (I had no idea what he actually said)—and I fell into a deep sleep.

Then, quite suddenly, I heard the command "Wake up." And I woke up without having the feeling of awakening out of a narcotic. I could not be astonished enough at this outcome.

IGNORING A CRISIS BRINGS A POSITIVE OUTCOME

In view of the special nature of the operation, I was required to lie on my back for several days without moving a muscle. Especially my head was not allowed to make the slightest movement. With the aid of sleeping tablets, and also taking into account the weakness of my heart, all movement was proscribed, making the days and nights immediately following the operation especially long.

Above all, I wasn't allowed to swallow since the fresh vocal chords needed to take root first. Intravenous nourishment became impossible after several days, since my veins were defending themselves against the needles. Both arms were swollen and sore.

The liver crisis feared beforehand by my doctor was indeed turning into reality. My excrement was spreading an incredible stench, and thus the women attendants were discharged and a male nurse took over.

When I tried for the first time to get up to use the bathroom on my own, I noticed a sharp stab in the region of my heart. I knew with certainty what that sharp pain meant—the presence of a severe heart condition that had appeared on every electrocardiogram taken up until that very day.

The computer monitoring my vital signs announced the truth immediately. And, the doctor who later looked after me, asked if I had known that I had suffered a serious heart attack. I told him that I was firmly convinced that by now Brother Death was on his way. I had wanted no disturbance around me at my death. For that reason, I said nothing at all about the heart attack.

My doctor thought that my very determination not to say anything probably had saved my life. For the absolute rest which I had wished for during the business of dying was also the best qualification for surmounting that crisis. ✳

AN ANTICIPATED REQUIEM

The doctors in Colleferro made a manifestly realistic judgment of the situation in spite of my silence about my heart condition. My chances of living were slim. As I learned later, there appeared in the world press an announcement: "Bernard Häring is about to die." In Africa, a translator's mistake arose, and the statement became "Father Häring has just died."

My former student, Bishop Michael Ntayahaga, celebrated in his cathedral in the capital city of Burundi, Bujumbura, a solemn requiem with a large attendance. This observance arose from his intention to solemnly admit his former tutor into African ancestry. No one has suffered any harm no matter what the intent of the prayer.

SICKNESS IS NOT GOD'S VENGEANCE

When I was again convalescent and out of immediate danger, I was given a copy of Milwaukee periodical called *The Wanderer*, originally a publication for German immigrants to the United States. This periodical routinely reflected very conservative views; and thus in it I read a long letter to the editor from an elderly priest. It was a hymn of praise to God who in his righteousness had at last chastened that old incorrigible sinner Bernard Häring.

My reaction was a feeling of deep sympathy for the old priest, coupled with a deep anxiety on account of the false notion of God which ever and again crops up in many a head and heart: a picture of God as avenger. Those who see God as punisher also seem to be members of a group whose mentality is such that they know with precision where the goats and where the sheep stand.

It reminds me of the personally shocking picture of the confessional director who wishes to know with precision the number and the species of every sin and directs the person to confess them in every detail.

My experience and the experiences of others tell us that often these "directing" types are ultimately the product of this notion of God which in the first place is directed against others. These are the same types who are also the ones subject to frightening anxieties.

I mention this experience for this reason only— that suffering in sickness and severe failure is seen by many people as unbearable because they and others think, and direct others to think, that their sickness and failures were decreed by an avenging God.

As for the judgment "God has punished him or her," if it is directed against some other objectionable person, this condemnation, objectively speaking, is one of the worst forms of the misuse of the name of God. ✻

SMOKERS AND
GOD'S WRATH

A gain and again, I have heard from people afflicted with cancer of the throat who have anxiously asked the question, "Why has the Creator punished me so severely for my habit of smoking?" My answer is one that always speaks from my own situation.

First of all, I draw attention to the fact that I myself was never a smoker. Every doctor who ever had anything to do with me during this sickness, and almost every nurse, asked me if I was a smoker. After my negative answer came the further question: "Did you live in a community with other smokers or talk often in smoky rooms?" To that question, I admit that I had to answer "yes."

All the same, I do not believe that smoking colleagues and smoky rooms were the chief cause of my illness. Instead, my illness was much more involved with psychosomatic factors.

If I had been a saint with perfect evenness of temper, the teaching investigation—which was chiefly concerned with the veto on speech—would have hit me less radically. I would have then been less vulnerable to the attack on my throat.

It was the teaching investigation and the fact that the Congregation of Faith expressed no compassion that resulted in greater pain than the actual physical crisis of health I suffered in Colleferro.

As a result, my main effort was concentrated on fighting against the feeling of bitterness and blame, not indeed with the idea of getting well again but rather with an eye toward a good death. Yet the overcoming of every bitterness may, in the long run, also have had something to do with my eventual recovery. God alone knows about that.

To smokers who see in their sickness a punishment directly from God, I say this: "I was not a smoker, and yet I have fallen ill. Many have smoked more than you and have not gotten cancer. There is no causal connection between smoking and God's punishment, even when smoking could be one of the causes of cancer."

"Yes, indeed," you might say, "doesn't the answer need to go deeper?" And I have often said and written: "God has not prescribed cancer for me." Cancer has to do with the world that has gotten into disorder. But God has given me grace and inner strength to inform the suffering with an acceptable meaning. That is an unmerited gift, but it also does require our cooperation.

In times of my sickness and with the feeling that Brother Death was close at hand, contemplation of the

Passion and the Resurrection of Christ meant more than ever to me. I could better feel my way into the heart of Jesus, filled as it is with sorrow and yet still overflowing with love. These sorrows give an acceptable meaning only if the Resurrection is kept in view.

I have found, in a special way, much consolation in the contemplation of the Letter to the Hebrews. "It was fitting that God, for whom and through whom all things exist, in bringing many children to glory, should make the pioneer of their salvation perfect through sufferings" (Hebrews 2:10).

"Because he himself was tested by what he suffered, he is able to help those who are being tested" (Hebrews 2:18).

In the Letter to the Hebrews, Jesus stands before us as one who is in a position to bear patiently with the ignorant and erring, since he, too, is beset by weakness (5:2). And, also, of Jesus it is said that he learned obedience and surrender in the school of suffering, as indicated in Hebrews 5:8. ✺

SUFFERING IS WORTH
THE TROUBLE

Though my Italian physician, Dr. Fratarcangelo, had never accepted a penny from me, he did ask me to do something for him in return. He told me how he had spent whole nights in a sweat when obliged to tell a patient that nothing more could be done to save his or her larynx. In this situation, one of these patients committed suicide, and two others attempted it.

Now, he tells his patients that he knows a priest who is also without a larynx and is happy all the time. (In the end I lost my larynx permanently.) His patients certainly must have thought that the good doctor was telling them a pious fib. It became quite a different story when I myself agreed to direct contact with the sick. One has quite a different charisma for consolation and encouragement when the rest of the sick know that you are speaking from experience. Here is one such story which shows the effect of such a direct approach.

Shortly before going on a trip to Rome, I received a brief note from a theological student. In it, she related that Hildegard Goss-Mayr, the great prophetess of nonviolence, had stated in a lecture that I was without a larynx and yet still enjoyed bearing witness to the Good News. The student's father was then faced with the total removal of his larynx, and he and her mother had begun to question their entire faith. "Help us," she pleaded.

Before my departure I wrote to the sick man and gave him an account of my faith experience in my own sickness. My letter to him arrived opportunely before his operation. And the addressee passed it on to his fellow patients.

Correspondence followed, and after that, came visiting. Unhappily, my friend was not so fortunate as I was. After four big operations, he suffered unspeakable pain which could scarcely be moderated. He wanted me to give him the sacrament of the sick.

This man was a cradle Catholic. I celebrated a Mass in his home—which was attended by his sister-in-law and her husband, recent settlers from Poland. Shortly before the war, her former husband, who had joined the Communists, left her because she wished to remain loyal to her faith.

Then she married a widower with young children. Notwithstanding these facts, her Polish diocese refused her a Declaration of Nullity of the first marriage. Both husband and wife went to confession and took part in the house Mass with much emotional involvement. Afterwards, my terminally ill friend said to me with astonishing calm: "My suffering was worth the trouble when I consider how happy these two are today."

After his death, his daughter wrote to me (meanwhile she had been raised to pastoral rank): "My father was a proud man. But he died a totally humble man." On such occasions, I thought many a time: "Even my suffering has paid rich dividends." ✤

RELAPSE: GRASPING
AT STRAWS

Professor Fratarcangelo, my physician, considered cobalt radiation necessary to full recovery. But the radiologist, who was completely astonished by my full, clear voice, asked him: "Do you really want us to burn your masterpiece in two?" So more numerous examinations took place instead of radiation therapy.

Two years passed relatively uneventfully. However, the Congregation of Faith still continued its teaching investigation and showed no anxiety over the fact that it could become partly to blame for a relapse.

Again I held my regular lectures and spent my long academic sabbaticals in the Third World charged with a variety of interesting duties. In 1979, when the teaching investigation was sinking into its last stages, I already felt signs of a relapse.

Once more, I experienced a game all too familiar to me. One simply does not wish to believe that one has cancer. One tries—despite all the signs—to crowd it out. The doctor speaks again of a polyp.

Secretly I thought to myself, "You poor fibber, you.

I know, of course, that I am going to lose my larynx since you, dear doctor, are in a bath of perspiration and can no longer sleep soundly." And yet I still went on clinging quite a while to this miserable wisp of straw-hope: a polyp. ✣

AND STILL: A THOUSAND REASONS FOR DANCING

Not only the psalmist but, above all, the Africans have taught me this: "And yet I wish to dance and sing." Though singing was admittedly out of the question, I reminded myself in all critical situations of my "key" dream, saying to myself, "I still have a thousand and more reasons for thanking God." My repeated prayer of thanksgiving was, it is true, weak and cold, as if it had come out of a monastery garden.

Then, after I had satisfied myself that no one saw me, I performed a dance for the dear God and for myself, so that the bodily expression of my gratitude should correspond more closely with my heart; that is, I had every reason for uninhibited gratitude.

To be sure, my dance was not especially artistic, but it was meant to be taken seriously. It wasn't only my body that warmed up. I also got warmer around my heart. The "nevertheless" of faith and gratitude carried the victory.

TRYING TO FEND OFF
THE INEVITABLE

In the late autumn of 1979, Dr. Fratarcangelo made yet another attempt to save my larynx by means of minor operations. However, a long strike of technical personnel caused a breakdown in an attempt to heal by heat through a short circuit through the neck. Strikes among workers in Italian nursing homes soon followed.

These events—coupled with my chronic liver trouble—created strong doubts about my undergoing another major operation. But, another postponement would have left me with little hope. So my doctor asked my superior in Rome to send me as quickly as possible to Germany where perhaps a German doctor may have other treatment options.

RESIGNATION

When the throat cancer was at the point of breaking through once more, I had just sent the first volume of my summary work of moral theology *Free and Faithful in Christ* in typescript to its American publishers. My work on the second volume had barely begun.

When I started this work in 1977, the thought as to whether the work would be brought to completion did not bother me at the time. Even the idea that it might never be completed did not bother me much at that point.

In 1979 and 1980, I felt otherwise, since the approach of death was highly probable. In the meanwhile, I had completed the second volume, and the first part of the third volume on bioethics.

The larger, more comprehensive and, for me, the harder part, *Healing of Public Life*, was hardly even sketched in outline. I regarded this final task as the culmination of my lifework, since *The Law of Christ* that had appeared in 1954 and which had been translated into several languages was, in my view, hopelessly out-of-date through the growth of historical consciousness and the work of the Second Vatican Council.

So, I had to resign myself to the thought that death would catch up with me before the completion of my life's work. I received a great deal of help in this matter of resignation from an experience of faith which I had undergone many years before. Since this experience may be helpful to others, I am recounting it here.

Dr. Brandhuber was a dear colleague of mine, a former professor of the New Testament, my confessor, and a good friend. One day, during a walk together, he said to me, "If God gives me one more year of health, two books about ancient Syrian Christology, which I have already worked on for twenty-five years, will be finished." Six months later, a cancer of the lung— already far advanced—was discovered.

Soon he was confined to bed and in need of continuing care. Since he sweated profusely and had to be dried out every two hours, I took my turn on the night shift as an assistant medical orderly.

Repeatedly, I tried to let my dear friend make a clean breast of his anxiety and discard his hope that God would still give him time to bring his life's work to a conclusion. It was just like an impenetrable wall between us whenever I wanted to go about making the situation clear to him.

One night, that situation suddenly altered. Once again I had changed his shirt and we were both tired from the effort. Then he beckoned to me to come closer. He had an important message to impart: "Now

I have grasped it. I long to be dissolved and to be with Christ." And for proof that he really had a complete grasp, he added: "Why now am I fretting about the material heaped up for my books?"

From that moment on, there was no more sweating. His countenance bore the mark of a deep peace. Perfectly relaxed, he awaited the great moment of his homecoming to Christ whom he had served so faithfully.

The thought that the work I had begun would never reach the end should really have affected me less deeply. For I had certainly made the body of my thought widely known. On the other hand, I was firmly convinced of the need for a new compendium of Catholic moral theology. If this compendium were to make a convincing and concise presentation of the progress made since the Second Vatican Council, then much systematic work still needed to be completed. The deeply gripping faith experience which Father Brandhuber had shared was of great assistance to me. It enabled me to hand over entirely to God's foresight the question of whether the work I had started would be brought to an end undisturbed. ❧

BOUNDLESS CONFIDENCE

With death approaching, the question of humanity became of much greater significance to me. This contemplation of humanity evolved into a consideration of the problem areas of the transmigration of souls, regeneration, and the Catholic teaching on purgatory.

Of what use was it for me to come before the Lord of life and death with my life as unfinished as a piece of patchwork? The answer, which I always gave myself anew when I was standing once more at the threshold of death, was made clear to me by a comrade, Francis Bourdeau, an early listener to, and outstanding translator of, my work *The Law of Christ*.

A few hours before his death, he wrote in a letter which lay on his table unfinished: "What happiness it is that in death we ought not to rely on anything we have done or services we have rendered, but solely on God's boundless goodness and grace."

In his final essay which he had sent shortly before his death for publication, he wrote with reference to purgatory: "There is no other fire than that of the love of God which purifies us and brings to perfection what is imperfect."

Another colleague, equally very dear to me, who has performed much generous service, Father Kurt-Dietrick Buche, offered me an appropriate word about dying which, frankly, had become for me a deadly serious issue. "Pray for me that I do not put the blame on God for my dying." He went on to clarify this statement: "When we die in a state of fear and anxiety, we dishonor our good God."

In this conversation about faith, we were both convinced also that the founder of our order had left us a precious saying in this regard: "It is not possible to honor God our Father better than by boundless confidence." ✻

DESPERATE MEASURES

Arriving in Germany to see if any help could be found there for my cancerous throat, I found that the doctors in charge of my medical care were already away on Christmas leave. I spent my waiting time in Kempten in the company of two Redemptorist Sisters.

There I decided to embark on a basic but radical cure: forty-two days of fasting—with a bottle of beet juice and much unsweetened tea for daily sustenance. This regime was for the purpose of cleansing my system.

Each day during this fast I took an hour's walk, gave much time over to prayer, and yet also worked for some hours on the third volume of my work on moral theology *Free in Christ*. At the very least, I wanted to sketch out a plan for how this work could be completed after my death.

After twenty days, I concentrated entirely on prayer and fasting, never giving up hope of starving the cancer by fasting. Colleagues had assured me that the red beet juice could in no way be assimilated by the cancer or drawn into it. And that turned out to be true.

As soon as I began to eat, however, the shrunken cancer again drew itself as much as it could, so that with all speed, the air-tube incision had to be dealt with first. ❧

THE SHARPEST SUFFERING
OF MY LIFE

This preliminary operation on my air-tube incision was performed by Dr. Westhues in a private nursing home. Since everything took place in a matter of minutes, it was not possible for an anesthetic to be administered beforehand. A choking sensation was constantly with me. As in 1977, an opening was made with the help of plastic, but the new air-tube opening seemed much more complicated.

Opposite me in the operating room was a crucifix. During the operation, I directed my gaze and my whole attention to the crucified Christ. Two nursing Sisters supported my arms. Each moment seemed like an eternity until finally I could snatch a breath through the new opening. Afterwards, the two nurses and the doctor complimented me on my iron discipline but, in truth, what else was there for me to do.

Afterwards there followed two weeks of preparation for the big operation—to which Dr. Westhues committed himself since he was quite certain that, through my fasting remedy, my liver had improved outstandingly. Even so, the anesthetist, who did not share my confidence in my beet-juice cure, showed great concern.

At our first meeting, I had told Dr. Westhues that I had lost my patience with pious fibs. He agreed with me that he would speak with complete frankness. And to him it was clear that my chances were minimal, since the cancer had advanced far beyond the area of the throat.

During my recovery period at both Colleferro and Starnberg, nurses looked after me far beyond their own proper time of duty. I cannot give them all sufficient praise for their efforts. For the first five nights after this operation, a nurse from Starnberg sat by my side. I had an immediate sense of her as a warm, compassionate presence. ⚘

VISITORS BRING SOLACE

The first visitor from the city of Starnberg was the evangelical pastor who brought me a magnificent bouquet of orchids from his wife. He had learned of my presence from a secretary of the parish, whose husband was in charge of the diet cooking.

The evangelical pastor presented himself as an old acquaintance since, years before, he had taken part in spiritual exercises I had conducted for the evangelical pastoral clergy and their wives. On the following day, he returned in the company of the city parish priest. This experience of ecumenicity alone was balm for my soul.

For sixteen days I was fed through a tube from my nose to my stomach, and this situation did not permit many visitors. My brothers, relations, and friends came as soon as visits were authorized.

Another steadfast visitor who came every day was Auxiliary Bishop Schmidt of Augsburg. Since I was over the worst, he celebrated Holy Mass every day in my sickroom in a manner so humanly moving and in such close proximity that for me these experiences were unforgettable.

With the roughest phase of my recovery behind me, Professor Westhues remarked that he still had something to talk over with me. When he spoke of this delayed conversation for a second time, I wrote on my bedside tablet: "I know what it is already. You wish to tell me that radiation is necessary."

Dr. Westhues breathed a sigh of relief. "Yes, that is it," he said, and proposed that I go to the Schwabinger nursing home, which was considered the best choice for this kind of treatment. I felt that, at the very least, I was quite over my temptation to create illusions about my illness. Or will one ever be quite clear of that temptation?

BREVITY IS THE SALT
OF LIFE

Each nun and nurse in turn came to receive the sacrament of reconciliation from me. The mystery of confession certainly had taken on a new form and meaning for me. Certainly I was silent, and I was learning more and more to speak with my eyes, in fact with the whole of my body, in place of a reliance on my voice.

Of course I had my writing tablet which I gladly and often used to answer questions or to convey a short message. I also used this tablet to give to those who came for confession an appropriate sentence, a word of joy, and a phrase of encouragement. And most admittedly I learned: "In brevity lies the salt of life." And, with the loss of the larynx and the windpipe, the temptation to gossip ceases. ✻

HEALING ENCOURAGEMENT: LEARNING TO SPEAK AGAIN

B efore the operation, Dr. Westhues told me that I would learn to speak again, but he did not explain how that would happen. He obviously took it for granted that I was aware of his decision that I learn to speak using my esophagus. But of this I was altogether uninformed.

Ten days after the surgery, a speech therapist arrived in my room. I still had the tube from my nose to my stomach, so our first visit was only a get-acquainted session.

The therapist gave me a book that covered directions for the study of esophageal speech, and she encouraged me to practice taking a couple of gulps of a carbonated beverage and to carefully observe the bubbling-up. On the phenomenon of the bubbling-up of stomach air is built the use of the food channel for renewed speech.

As soon as the feeding tube was removed, I tried to make a sound with the bubbling-up of stomach air. And, just look at it! I had the knack of it almost at once! When, a couple of days later, three of my own flesh-

and-blood sisters came to see me, I spoke to each close by her ear. They were beside themselves with astonishment, for they had been convinced that I was going to remain dumb for the rest of my life.

At the invitation of Dr. Westhues, I was visited twice by an elderly teacher from Munich who had lost his larynx. He had had the operation fifteen years prior to me, but it was more than five years later that he had learned to speak by means of using his food passage. He even sang a short song for me. For several years, he visited everyone in the Munich area who had been recently operated on for the removal of the larynx.

I also later became acquainted with a lady who visited every woman in the Munich area who had suffered this loss as well. Both did this as a matter of an innermost urging. Not once did they allow themselves to be reimbursed for traveling expenses. They were the very embodiment of the solidarity of those who suffer.

When the speech therapist visited me in Starnberg the second time, she was speechless to find that I could actually speak some syllables. She told me that when she had first met with Dr. Westhues, he had said with great discernment, "Don't dare to offer Professor Häring an electronic appliance. The man has enough intelligence and skill to use his esophagus for speech." That is a brilliant example of healing encouragement, so different from moralizing.

Madam Fuchs had been recommended to me at the nursing home in Starnberg as a speech therapist. She was a very big help to me. On her first visit, she wanted to know how far I wished to learn this art, and I was able to tell her immediately, even though with broken hesitation, that I wanted to learn to speak well enough to celebrate the Eucharist in a fitting manner and to proclaim the Good News again. I thought I could tell from her eyes her opinion of the elderly man who quite plainly was wishing to undertake too much.

Madam Fuchs understood in grand style how to give encouragement. For example, when I did not bring out the letter "f" plainly, she said: "That sound we can simply leave alone. Later it will come right by itself."

In this strategy I can see an example for the teaching of moral theology. Instead of tying ourselves down to strict imperatives, we can and should look at the common law of growth. Everything has its proper time, and it is important that we are all together on the way.

One day Madam Fuchs told me that a mother of several children who waited with me every day for radiation treatments, could not bring herself to speak even one word in the waiting area, for she felt ashamed of the male-sounding voice coming out of her esophagus. Madam Fuchs was convinced that this woman would have no inhibitions in my presence. So we conducted our daily speech exercises with Madam

Fuchs together, and with that arrangement, the problem was solved.

After having had a series of fifteen radiation treatments, the business of correction was undertaken. Because of dryness of the mouth and in the esophagus, it would always be more difficult to bring a sound out. After thirty-five radiation treatments, my speech faculty was once more immobilized. After two months, however, I was able to resume my speech practice.

In all, I met with Madam Fuchs twenty-five times, some ten minutes at a time. After the last practice, Madam Fuchs asked me to give her an opportunity to talk about her faith. This conversation lasted about an hour. Then, as she congratulated me, she said: "Now you are so advanced that you can again celebrate the Eucharist and proclaim the Good News." ✻

INCONCEIVABLE JOY IN SPEAKING ONCE MORE

M adam Fuchs also advised me to follow a continuing course of speech therapy in Nurnberg which had the best speech trainers in Europe. A whole group of young speech therapists were together—some for advanced study and others were beginners.

This course was richly rewarding to me. When I started with Madam Fuchs, the Ruktus method was the only one I knew anything about. This method consists of taking a gulp of air with which you bring out two to four syllables. With the Ruktus method, you can speak only haltingly, and the use of a microphone is impossible since with every new gulp of air the microphone crackles.

Slowly and with some difficulty, I was able to change over to the method of uninterrupted inhaling of air. With the ongoing course, I made great progress. While speaking, one is constantly taking in air which, with a suckling motion like taking in mother's milk, the air flows through the food tube into the stomach and without interruption flows back again. The voice is formed on the upper rim of the food tube.

On the evening before the course began, I sat at table with a younger woman who had been operated on three years before, but she had never, up to this point, uttered a sound.

After her operation, this woman had, like myself, been given radiation treatments, and since she was pregnant, she was advised to have her pregnancy interrupted. She declined, and the child she bore was lame. At that, her husband left her. Fortunately, she had a good mother who took care of the child so that she could return to work to support herself and her child.

A speech therapist from Luxembourg took a special interest in this young woman. Three days later, she was able to say on the telephone to her mother: "Mother, I can speak," to the inconceivable joy of both.

During the course I got to know yet another woman who likewise was pregnant when she was given radiation treatments. She also categorically refused to have her pregnancy interrupted, and she gave birth to a healthy child.

This woman, however, had the total support of her husband. The child, who was then about three years of age, understood her mother's voice perfectly, although it was unintelligible to the rest of us, including her husband. This woman was taken in hand by the best speech therapist in Holland who, with a colleague, had developed the use of the artificial esophagus voice some thirty years before.

It has now been nearly thirteen years since I learned how to use the artificial esophagus voice. Without any difficulty, I can hold three or four lectures a day. (The provision of a good microphone is, of course, taken for granted.) ✻

RELYING ON MYSELF: MORE RADIATION

It was abundantly clear to Dr. Westhues and the radiation specialist that I would need the highest amount of radiation permissible for the course of my thirty-five radiation treatments. It was my great good fortune that the leading tomographer in Munich was available in private practice. The Schwabinger radiation center sent me to this specialist.

Millimeter by millimeter, the tomographer evaluated the situation so that the radiologist, by means of this evaluation, would know exactly where and how strongly the radiation ought to be applied. I am convinced that his innovative approach saved my life. For without the talents of the tomographer, the thirty-five radiation treatments would have largely been expended to no purpose.

The very sympathetic radiologist drew my attention, as he was duty bound, to all the effects of the radiation to be anticipated: "You will in all probability lose all your teeth and very likely all your hair as well. Your mouth will suffer from great dryness. Your sense of taste will be dead for some time, and so on."

Then he said to me, "Nearly all your fellow sufferers are always looking for stronger sleeping medication and painkillers. I believe that you can basically rely on yourself to renounce all the stronger sleeping medication."

I recall precisely his formula: "You can rely on yourself." For me, that is a classic expression of the charismatic way of speaking encouragement which addresses itself to the deepest interior sources of strength. This approach is radically different from moralism, which merely orders people around. As a result, I really did rely on myself and stood up to the thirty-five cobalt treatments significantly better than those who took strong pain-killing medication.

While undergoing radiation treatment, I lived in the Redemptorist monastery in Munich. There a missionary sister from Gars cooked easily digestible food for me and encouraged me to eat enough, even though every kind of food tasted the same after all the cobalt treatments. It took a good year until my sense of taste gradually began to function again.

My approach to this experience was a great moral duty which must be done without a feeling of self-satisfaction. Now I am better able to understand the passage from Friedrich Schiller on the Kantian moral rule: "Gladly am I of service to friends, yet also, I do it out of inclination, and so it grieves me much that I am not virtuous. On this matter no other advice is useful other than to despise and carry out what duty bids."

How glad I was when I could again routinely relish the good flavor of food. At the same time, the saliva glands started to function again. On the other hand, my sense of smell remained out of action, for the simple reason that I do not breathe through the nose but am a chest breather.

Still I can say that I have plenty of joy in life, in all things beautiful and good; yes, even in my miserable artificial esophagus voice. I see in this a great gift of God. I have in these years given many lectures and exercises and conducted numerous services of healing. To every "if and but," I have bidden farewell and can say that I am fortunate in my way of life.

I cover the time of these thirty-five radiation treatments in depth because I did not concentrate on myself during this period, but rather on others and on my duty. I worked for some four hours daily on the last volume of my work *Free in Christ.* I wrote this last work out in longhand since in my situation typewriting might have provided increasing difficulties because of my drainage tube. Moreover, dictation, which I practiced before on a large scale, was out of the question since my artificial voice could not take the place of a dictating voice.

THE FELLOWSHIP OF
SUFFERING

In the basement of the Schwabinger nursing home, we often waited a long time for treatment—each one taking our turn. In this situation a genuine friendship slowly grew. Most of us were more or less silent like me. We developed a body language for communicating, laughing with one another and offering gestures of encouragement.

Waiting along with us grownups was a whole group of children whose radiation treatments were not directed toward the throat but to tumors in the brain. All of them except a nine-year-old child were accompanied by relatives. When this youngster saw that he had to wait like one forsaken, he cried bitterly. I tried to comfort him. From then on, he always came straight to me, nestled close beside me, and shed his tears on my sleeve. By degrees he came to feel so comforted that he found weeping no longer necessary.

A man my own age who had a cancer on the tongue made it clear to me that he was thinking about committing suicide. At that I began to write a timely note for everyone who was waiting with me for radiation. I saw that my brief notes were treasured. Many waited purposely for them. One day there appeared among us in the basement waiting for cobalt radiation a woman in a wheel chair. She gave every one of us a friendly smile. To her also I wrote a note: "Your delightful smile here in the basement is worth more than a million marks." She received my little note with a friendly encouraging laugh.

All in all, I regard the experience in the radiation cellar of the Schwabinger nursing home as one of the most precious enrichments of my life. When I had the first checkup with my doctor in Rome, he said to me, "The work which Dr. Westhues has done for you is an unsurpassed master achievement. And the same is true for the radiation center at Munich."

GOD HELPS YET AGAIN

Right after the six-hour operation in the Starnberg clinic, Dr. Westhues told my superiors, "I do not believe that I have succeeded in uncovering every nest of cancer and clearing it out." He had stuck fast to my previous request not to indulge in any white lies.

Only after a basic checkup three years after the big operation did Dr. Westhues abandon his reserve and say, "God has helped us once again." I answered spontaneously, "Yes, through your competency and concern." And this was his answer: "That I cannot accept. For that we must give the honor to God."

Spontaneously there came to me the remembrance of what Professor Fratarcangelo had said in 1977 before the previous five-hour operation took place: "If God helps us." It is at once astonishing and cheering that these two great men of action straightaway give God the honor as a matter of course and commend themselves to him for help. ✺

ANOTHER RELAPSE—AND A MIRACULOUS REMISSION

If the cancer has shown no further sign of revival after six years, then according to professional pronouncements you have a high degree of certitude that you have escaped from the evil of this disease; that is, you are definitely healed. That is the optimism I felt five or six years after the big operation in Starnberg: fully certain. I was so certain that I no longer went for checkups; and I had the feeling that I would come out of this battle for health without the aid of a doctor.

But just as I was lulled into complacency, a strong rash appeared around the skin near the incision in my throat. After a few days, the whole of my chest looked like a scab.

I went to our house doctor in Salvator Mundi, to a good well-furnished nursing home of German Sisters. After the basic checkup, the doctor obliged my request for a complete explanation of all the results. I wasn't surprised when I read the results of the cardiogram: "The test indicates a serious heart condition," since troubles with my heart went back almost ten years.

Then I read: "Lung expanded by about a third,

pressing on the heart, and fully occupied by double-headed knots." I noticed immediately that the Italian name for these knots corresponded exactly with the name of the cancer of the larynx. The doctor had told me at the time that this special form of cancer is particularly obstinate.

I knew where I stood. I told myself that at my age the process of disease doesn't run all that swiftly, so that it was possible I still had time to see my last doctoral candidates through to the end. Certainly one thing was clear: I had to get myself ready in earnest for the visit of Brother Death.

The doctor prescribed a medicine which contained cortisone, but in small doses. The label indicated that this medicine ought not to be prescribed for old people, but if it were, only in quite small doses. In keeping with the description on the label, this drug was expected to promote the slowing down of the progress of the sickness.

Even so, my doctor handed me over to the best cancer specialist in Rome. My Superior General advised me to go to Germany in the hope of finding an even better doctor there. I decided to stay in Rome. I thought that I could hardly find a greater expert, and at my age it is certainly normal to think of death. He accepted this answer; and I endeavored to cultivate a deeper life of prayer, but also carried on with my usual jobs, although I was feeling rather wretched.

After some months, the clinical practitioner carried out anew a thorough-going checkup. I was not a little astonished when he shared the result with me: "The cancer knots are all in a state of total decay." My reaction was: "I should like to believe it. But it sounds too good to be believable. Could you, as a doctor, explain that to me?"

After a thoughtful start he referred to interior sources of healing power that scientifically were hardly comprehensible. Finally, I asked him yet again, would he, please, explain, as far as possible in scientific terms, because it still appeared to me incomprehensible. At that he looked in his drawer for quite a while, drew from it a Jesus picture and in reference to it said only: "I believe in Him." Not another word about the cause. The scablike inflammation on the chest went away relatively quickly.

When, in April 1988, I finally took leave of Rome, I received a visit from my doctor and his wife. He told me before leaving: "Your healing was a miracle" without adding anything else.

Naturally, I have reflected a great deal about this. I cannot make much sense of the notion of a miracle as an annulment of the laws of nature. I am thinking of a kind of peak experience of a spiritual nature which, like a spark, can jump across the powers of body and soul.

At all events I drew the one sure conclusion: to

thank God always and above all, and to put all my trust in him. Our first and foremost concern ought not to be about our health but about doing the will of God and the coming of his kingdom. With that, all the rest will be given us.

Now I can say once again: God has not prescribed cancer for me. But he has granted me light and strength to live with it purposefully and to fight against the sickness. ✤

MEDICINE PROLONGS MY LIFE
YET ONCE MORE

Immediately after my return from Rome to Gars, I was forced to go into the hospital for an operation for a rupture of the groin. Not once did I allow them to give me the anointing of the sick, although I had permitted this prior to all my previous operations. I regarded this operation as a small matter. I was all the more surprised when it took more than four hours to complete this operation. When I came back from the operating room, I felt totally miserable. The long-lasting narcotic had exhausted me beyond my usual limits. But now the question arose: what actually happened?

On the next day, Dr. Bauer, the principal doctor who had performed the operation with the help of one assistant, sat down on the edge of my bed and said: "There is still one serious matter to be mentioned. During the operation, which was a thoroughly disagreeable affair, I wondered whether an artificial bowel outlet should be made at once. [Editor's note: The construction of an artificial opening from the colon through the abdominal wall, consequently bypassing a diseased segment of the lower intestine and permitting the passage of intestinal contents, is called a colostomy in surgical language.] That is the question before us now."

I took this news with outward calm. But when I was alone in prayer I cried: "Dear God, already I have an artificial entrance for air, and now, added to this, an artificial bowel outlet: isn't this too much for one weak mortal?"

The question about the bowel outlet still hung in the air when suddenly I fell into a high fever. A lung X-ray was taken to make sure that everything in that regard was in order.

Next, when Dr. Bauer tore the dressing from the wound with some force, a yellow spot, a sign of an infection, appeared in the pit of the stomach. Since a narcotic was no longer thinkable after the experience of the groin operation, the pus had to be squeezed out twice a day, with a fair amount of force, without any anesthetic.

Dr. Bauer said to me: "You may rest assured, I know of no other way." The pus flowed away at last in great measure. For four days round the clock I persevered with antibiotics. It was clear to me that it was only because of the unheard developments of science that I still had a chance of life.

Again I must praise the outstandingly devoted and competent attention to duty on the part of the nurses.

The caring style of this kind of duty is also a means of healing and one of the highest importance.

When I was discharged from the hospital, the chief doctor came to see me himself. This is what he said in front of the nuns and the doctor in charge: "Father Häring is a master of the art of concealing pain."

Indeed, what else could I do? In my situation, as one without a throat larynx, I couldn't cry out at all, even if I had wanted to.

I recovered at an astonishing speed. I started again to take long walks, stayed in the consulting room for the benefit of the many who were seeking advice, again held lectures, and wrote essays meant to show that where my health was concerned, everything was working out for the best. ✳

DIVINE DISPENSATION

In the course of the summer of 1989 my humanity made itself known with full force through the occurrence of some brain seizures. One of them began during sleep, and threw me out of bed. I had the sensation of an enormous earthquake, as if my bed were revolving, and the whole room was standing on its head. When after some time I came back fully to myself, I turned on the light and was not a little astonished that no books had fallen down and everything stood in its proper place.

I cannot yet understand even today, why, after this experience, I did not go straight to the doctor. It was while I was standing in for the parish priest in my own home district that the next strong brain seizure befell me, and after that, I did seek the advice of a doctor.

This doctor put his finger at once on the right diagnosis. Because of the healing of the wounds on my throat in the wake of many operations and numerous radiation treatments, the blood circulation to my brain became all the more imperfect.

I was directed to a neurologist, who understandably was afraid there could also be a brain tumor developing. According to the brain scan, however, this was not the case. However, the scan did show the extent of the true cause: an inadequate supply of blood to both halves of the brain. Stronger medicine—as well as stronger tranquilizers—were needed to meet the onset of renewed brain seizures. I regarded these medicines as a worthwhile reserve supply.

In December of 1989, a brain seizure hit me like a thunderstorm. Then, later in the afternoon came a whole series of brain seizures. By the evening I was given the anointing of the sick. I, as well as the priest who anointed me, thought that death was appreciably near. In the midst of this expectation, I lost consciousness, and at this point the neurologist appeared. He gave me a series of electric shocks as he later explained. It was a risk which was probably able to sidetrack immediate death. And, it certainly achieved what was hoped for, even if it did not result in an all-around surer improvement. By the next day I was again quite conscious.

In this dangerous situation, I experienced once again a favorable gift of divine foresight. Others may describe it as a happy accident. In my opinion, however, it follows more easily, even from the standpoint of mere reason, to speak of a dispensation of divine providence rather than to call it a pure accident.

When my sister, Lucidia Häring, who was in charge of a school for those who have care of the sick and had connections with a large hospital, heard of my illness, she telephoned my Superior with the message that the doctor might do well to investigate the function of the adjoining thyroid gland. She had experience with many patients whose brain seizures resulted from a lack of calcium. My Superior brought me her message at once.

Then, just as I was leaving my room, I happened to meet Dr. Englert, a doctor of outstanding distinction, who had been visiting another patient in the hospital. He greeted me as a friend and asked how I was. I, for my part, took advantage of the situation to ask if my sister's judgment was useful. He affirmed it and at that point, I asked him to accept me as a patient. Without delay, he arranged a thorough examination.

This examination showed that not only had the adjoining thyroid gland made a notable contribution to my seizures, but that the gland itself was close to useless. Along with all that, my blood values were also in a state of chaos.

Dr. Englert consulted a thyroid-gland specialist in Munich. In astonishment, this specialist said: "With these results rarely is the patient still alive."

Because of my serious heart condition and present crisis, the artificial thyroid gland hormones had to be introduced in a creepingly slow manner. In order to treat the blood supply to the brain, the doctor ordered an immediate changeover to an extract from the Chinese ginkgo tree, a medication which showed excellent results.

In spite of this, however, as each day passed, my paralysis of apoplectic origin was getting worse. [Editor's note: A blockage or hemorrhage of a blood vessel leading to the brain, causing inadequate oxygen supply, resulting in a sudden, usually marked loss of bodily function as in a stroke.] For this reason, all tranquilizers had to be set aside. The consequence of this was total sleeplessness accompanied by hallucinations.

Since I could neither read nor pray my breviary, I had to rely much more on the cultivation of the already long-loved Abba prayer—a prayer which, here and now, I would like to recommend to sick and well alike. Even Dr. Englert surmised that it had contributed to what was to him a simply inexplicable healing. With the onset of my blood seizures, my blood values were chaotic; one year later, my blood values reached the ideal, and in the words of Dr. Englert "a twenty-year-old could not wish for better." Moreover, the paralysis was, by this time, fully overcome. Since then I have been able to work like a much younger man.

THE LOVING FATHER
PROVIDES AID AGAIN

"If we live, we live to the Lord, and if we die, we die to the Lord" (Romans 14:8). I wrote these optimistic words about my health in the spring of 1993. Indeed another six full months of health and happy apostolic activities followed. Then, at the end of September, optimism about health yielded its place to the need for enormous hope.

On Sunday, September 26, after a sleepless night, I tried to get up around four o'clock in the morning, but fell back on the bed with an enormous storm of brain convulsions. I felt that these convulsions arose from below and pervaded my entire brain. This lasted for more than three hours.

There was no possibility of calling anyone to help since I was completely immobilized. So, I called upon the Lord. I thought about his abandonment on the cross for the space of three hours, and then I concentrated all my attention on the last prayer of Jesus as he hung on the cross: "Father, into your hands I commend my spirit" (Luke 23:46). I watched my breath, waiting for the moment in which I would commit my last breath into the hands of the loving Father. When death seemed to be so close at hand, nothing could weaken my determination to conform myself with Jesus in His loving trust in His Father.

At seven o'clock in the morning, a nun arrived at the monastery to call me for Sunday Mass. So, beyond all my expectations, they found me, still conscious. The Superior celebrated with me the sacrament of anointing and gave me absolution.

The brain convulsions were still continuing when the doctor arrived. Happily, he knew at once what kind of injection could stop them, so I continued to cling to life. This time however, I had no optimism for a full or nearly full recovery.

A thorough-going diagnostic examination found the main cause of these renewed brain seizures: grave damage of the cervical vertebrae, most probably as a consequence of the radiation therapy received more than thirteen years ago, a side effect worth accepting after so many good years.

Since then, good doctors and an outstanding physiotherapist have done everything to make my life acceptable: thanks be to God! How privileged I am, above all, for the gift of faith and trust in God, and then for the loving care which I receive so abundantly.

Every hour I live is precious if I follow the vision of Saint Paul, living to the Lord and dying to him as well. In terms of the suffering which is unavoidable in these circumstances, I find great consolation in the words of Charles De Foucauld: "If in conformity with Jesus Christ we suffer patiently, then we may have great confidence that our prayer of love of God is authentic." ✻

PART II

The Healing Power of the Abba-Father

HIDDEN IN *HIM*

I believe there is no greater healing power than the hidden knowledge of the self found in the grace of the Abba-Father, the knowledge that the wholly good Savior has lovingly accepted one's own self, and the inspiration of the Holy Spirit which leads to self-animation and the freedom to take the initiative.

We ought to consider with what limitless love and respect Jesus approached the sick and presented them with an unmerited payment of trust in advance of friendship. This is the point of view from which we must try to understand his miracles of healing.

As I have already said, I cannot imagine them as miracles brought about by an external power in re-settlement against the laws of nature. Rather all body/soul powers—and these are miraculous works of the Creator-Spirit in themselves—are aroused and brought together to the point when the spark of the Spirit catches fire, a spark that goes out from Jesus and the Father. In this way, the hidden powers of healing can be set free and raised to inconceivable heights.

And standing there in the background is the daily and sometimes astonishingly great experience of love which has been bestowed on us by our fellow men and women. It is there and by that means that God is also at work: "Where love and goodness are, there is God."

God the Creator is in all things. Certainly the most outstanding thing is the power of his love which shows itself discernible and efficacious in healing and curing interpersonal relationships and in communal and wholly personal experiences. ✤

THE ABBA-FATHER BREATH
OF JESUS

One way of experiencing all this power and letting it become efficacious is the Abba-Father Breath of Jesus. This means nothing less than allowing oneself to be consoled and fulfilled by this Abba-Father Breath of Jesus.

Our natural breath is a basic symbol of the love breath of God, of the Holy Spirit. The Hebrew word *rûah*, like the Greek word *pneuma* in the Bible, is usually translated as "breath." The Holy Breath, the Holy Spirit, is the eternal basic event of the breath of life and love between the Father and the Son. In the breath of their love, they are presenting themselves to each other from eternity in a state of unspeakable blissful affection.

Incidentally, in Hebrew both these expressions which refer to the Holy Breath of God (namely Breath and Wisdom) are feminine, an expression of motherly tenderness and fruitfulness.

The prayer of Jesus, in which the expression of inward love and total trust—Abba (Papa, dear heart, Father)—is quite central, should in the fulfillment of the Abba-Father prayer of Jesus constitute our breath, our life, and our love of it. It is thoroughly understandable that we would experience our breathing in and out as a basic symbol of our ability to let ourselves be grasped by the love of Jesus for the Father and for us.

When the disciples of Jesus came back, radiant with joy after their first mission to preach salvation and heal the sick, Jesus rejoiced in the holy Breath and said: "I thank you, Father, Lord of heaven and earth, because you have hidden these things from the wise and the intelligent and have revealed them to infants (Luke 10:21). ✺

WHEN YOU PRAY

When the disciples of Jesus experienced the Abba-Father prayer with wonder and astonishment, they asked him if he would teach them to pray. And what did he do? He took them straight into the Our Father (Luke 11:2), making them into one big family of his Father.

When Jesus prays and takes us up into his prayer, he is revealing himself in the history of salvation as the One Who Is From Eternity. As Thomas of Aquin says: He is "not any word but the Word which breathes love." The breath of love proceeds from the Father and goes out from him.

In the great eucharistic prayer at the evening supper before his departure, Jesus begins six times with "Abba." And he rejoices, "I have made your name known to those whom you gave me" (John 17:6).

In each of the six Abba-Father paragraphs of the high priestly prayer of Jesus, there emerges the happy thought that Jesus has received us as a gift from the Father and rejoices in the fact that we, his disciples, acknowledge that the Father himself has given his beloved Son to us as Redeemer and Friend. Constantly in the prayer of Jesus there recurs the theme of our being taken up into the eternal love between Father and Son in the Holy Breath, in the life and breath of love.

The Apostle Paul makes it explicit in three places that the Holy Breath of God himself takes us up into the Abba-Father prayer of Jesus.

God's love has been poured into our hearts through the Holy Spirit.

Romans 5:5

You have received a spirit of adoption. When we cry, "Abba! Father!" it is that very Spirit bearing witness with our spirit that we are children of God.

Romans 8:15-16

And because you are children, God has sent the Spirit of his Son into our hearts, crying, "Abba! Father!"

Galatians 4:6

There is a passage in the Letter to the Romans that for sick people and the severely tried carries a quite outstanding message of comfort and support:

Likewise the Spirit helps us in our weakness; for we do not know how to pray as we ought, but that very Spirit intercedes with sighs too deep for words. And God, who searches the heart, knows what is the mind of the Spirit, because the Spirit intercedes for the saints according to the will of God.

Romans 8:26-27 ✴

PAYING ATTENTION TO
YOUR BREATH

God, the *I-am-there*, "formed man from the dust of the ground, and breathed into his nostrils the breath of life; and the man become a living being" (Genesis 2:7). In this biblical view and prior to the Abba-Father prayer, we observe with ever-renewed gratitude our breath as a gift from the Creator and as a symbol of the three-in-one love of God.

And so, consider your breath as a symbol and copy of the Abba-Father Breath of Jesus. Let yourself be caught in the grip of an ever-growing astonishment that your breath can be to you a reminder that you yourself are totally taken up into the Breath of the everlasting love between the Father and Son.

Our breathing should be deep, gentle, and regular. Breathe out deeply and rest for a couple of seconds in the thought that with every breath you are entrusting yourself to God in order to find in him rest, and joy, and peace. *Ab* and *ba*.

With the intake of breath (at the first *Ab*), we experience ourselves as a gift that comes from the Father. We open ourselves to the constantly joyous experience of being as sons and daughters of God. With the outgoing of breath (at the *ba* of *Abba*), we give ourselves back to God with gratitude and trust. As for the pause between breathing out and breathing in, this we experience as being "hidden in him."

Let us be caught up in astonishment. Let us make room for joy. With that, the pauses between breathing out stale breath and taking in fresh will gradually become longer. By this means, the intake of breath will then become deeper with the experience of our dependence on God's love and breath of life.

GIVING YOURSELF TO
THE BREATH OF GOD

With Jesus, in the strength of his love, we may say: "Abba! Father in heaven!" Through the Abba-Father Breath of Jesus to which we give ourselves totally, we are, so to speak, in heaven. We are taken up completely into the inner divine giving between the Father and the Son through their own love-breath.

So with amazement and happiness, we give our praise inwardly with Jesus "the Lord of heaven and earth." If we name the Father in heaven trustingly with Jesus—Abba!—then that is a prayer that gives praise.

———— ✼ ————

Abba, may your name Abba be hallowed,
praised, and loved!
This great longing that the Father-Name of God be known, loved, and honored by all, belongs essentially to the Abba-Father prayer. It is there that a great power of healing lies.

In this prayer our basic purposes will be united. We

will become more sensitive about showing honor to the holy name of God, the Father of Our Lord Jesus Christ.

Our sickness and sufferings can no longer enslave us if, in union with Jesus through our Abba-Father prayer, our longing grows that the Father-Name of God be praised and loved on earth as it is in heaven. By degrees, we experience a sense of liberation from the narrowness of our small being, that our prayer, our life, our suffering, our love, if united to Jesus, will have endless value.

—— ✹ ——

Abba Father, thy kingdom come,
on earth as it is in heaven.

Jesus has lived and suffered among us in order to show us the Father, so as to take us up into his kingdom of love, grace, and peace, as men and women who are accepted as coworkers. Let us pause as we say our Abba-Father prayer for one, two, or three minutes to allow the longing for the coming of God's kingdom to grow strong in us. Then, with that, will also grow our longing to cooperate with it, not the least through self-abandonment and trust in God in days of sickness.

—— ✹ ——

Abba Father, thy will be done,
on earth as it is in heaven.

The Abba-Father prayer, faithfully practiced, gives us an inkling of heaven, of being taken up into the salvific plan of God by means of his inner divine blessedness and love overflowing to each of us. In the Abba-Father prayer, we are looking anew with astonishment at the prayer of Jesus on the Mount of Olives:

"Abba Father, thy plan of salvation, thy will be done, not mine."

The final, outgoing breath of Jesus on the Cross was his final "yes" to the salvific plan of the Father, the highest glorification of the Father-Name of God by means of unlimited trust. "Abba Father, into thy hands I commend my breath."

When sickness, suffering, and disillusionment are overpowering, are getting us down, we lift our attention to Jesus on the Cross and let ourselves be taken up by the love-breath of Jesus into his prayer: "Abba Father, into thy hands I commend myself, my life, and my last breath."

If the first part of the Our Father is the big existential step beyond the narrowness of the ego to the Thou of God, of his kingdom and of his plan of salvation, then the second part of the Our Father takes us in a special way right into salvation, solidarity with Jesus, who is all things to all of us, and teaches us to become all things to all of us, and teaches us to become free of egoism, whether individual or collective.

— ※ —

Abba, our Father,
give us this day our daily bread.
How costly is the bread which we gratefully receive from the hands of our loving Father! He gives us his beloved Son Jesus as the bread for the life of the world.

As long as we hand ourselves over to the Abba-Father Breath of Jesus earnestly, we can value everything we have received from God as his gift, as a sign of his Father-Love for us, but also for everyone. But if it is only my bread I am seeking, my honor, my success, then everything will have a bad taste. From out of the gift of the Abba-Father there will be a theft.

All of the gifts intended for us in general will then become prison chains of self-centeredness, and an occasion for envy, strife, violence, cheating, and war. The more our Abba-Father Name is the soul of our breath, our thoughts, and our dress, so much more easily do we step into the healing solidarity that comprises all earthly goods and every grace. A mighty power of sharing and community goes out from the Abba-Father Name.

— ※ —

Father, our Father, forgive us our guilt
as we also forgive all who are guilty of anything
against us.

The healing power of prayer is for me a central result of a realistic trust in God during sickness. We should direct with full intensity our loving gaze and attention to the prayer of Jesus on the Cross: "Abba Father, forgive them, for they do not know what they are doing."

Here again the astonishment with which we let ourselves be gripped has a higher meaning. It is not self-evident that Jesus on the Cross is praying to his beloved Father from his inmost heart for his torturers and for those who insulted him. It is my opinion that through his wounds, through his utterly uncompelled freedom from hostility, we are healed.

Gratitude, astonishment! Then will the forgiveness, the freedom from all bitterness and all rancor become to some extent self-evident. Certainly there still remains grace, a gift for which we must always renew our gratitude. And, if at any time, bitterness gets us in its clutches, then we pray the Abba-Father Breath Prayer with our gaze directed to Jesus on the cross, and at the same time, listen to his prayer from the heart: "Abba Father! Forgive!"

——— �֍ ———

Abba Father, let us not slide into temptation,
but set us free from evil.

These two petitions belong together. The temptation that matters above all others is the temptation to fall away from the kingdom of love and of peace and to give way to envy, hatred, and vindictiveness.

On the positive side, it is a request for the inward strength and health to avoid hostility. Jesus has loved me, a poor sinner, without limit and does not cease to love me, so that I also can love those who (apparently) have done me wrong. In the Abba-Father Breath Prayer say always more firmly: "Yes" to the advice: "Do not be overcome by evil, but overcome evil with good" (Romans 12:21).

— ✣ —

Abba Father! Amen! Yes, so be it.
That is what I hope for from your love.
I entrust myself to you forever. Amen.

Those who in the heartfelt offering of the Abba-Father Prayer let themselves be completely gripped by the Abba-Father Breath of Jesus, know that they are reconciled with God and will be taken into his reconciling healing action. That means a great deal for sick persons themselves, for the course of their illnesses, for their meaning, and lastly, for their final redemption. It means a great deal also for the salvation of the world.

Since many sick people are sometimes glad to have a set form of prayer, I am offering here several short prayers.

—— ✳ ——

IN THE MORNING I

I cry aloud to the LORD,
>and he answers me from his holy hill.
I lie down and sleep;
>I awake again, for the LORD sustains me.

Psalm 3:4-5

Abba! Father of the light! The darkness of this night has not disturbed me so very much, for you always let me feel afresh that you are beside me.

Yes, you are for me the *Here-I-am*.

In your fatherly care, I feel myself safely hidden, even if I awake from a disturbing dream. The Abba-Father Breath of your beloved Son brings me a gift of rest and peace, even at a time when sleep escapes me. Your breath of love flows through me, strengthens and consoles me.

Father! I thank you for the grace of faith, for the experience of trust, for the gift of your love. The more I feel strengthened by the Abba-Father prayer, so much so am I overcome by a deep feeling of sympathy with the sick and the aged, who either do not know you at all or see in you at the very most the judge. They may have doubts about your fatherly love, and for this reason: That in their lives, and more particularly in their sufferings, too little love from the heart was given them.

Have mercy on them. Send them this day and every day men and women who, through their goodness, their mutual feeling, and their readiness to help, let them have an inkling that you, God of love, are the very heart of all being. Help me this day to pass on to the men and women whom I meet something of the love and peace that you give me.

Amen ✳

IN THE MORNING II

I believe that I shall see the goodness of the LORD
   in the land of the living.
Wait for the LORD;
   be strong, and let your heart take courage;
Wait for the LORD!

Psalm 27:13-14

Abba, Father of love! The warm light of morning and the fresh air in the room give me a foretaste of the happily blessed awakening after my final intake of breath, after my last Abba-Father prayer. If I have breathed out my last breath on earth with trust in Jesus who, as in life and in death, has entrusted himself wholly to you; yes, if I awaken to a life full, new, and lasting, then shall I look upon your face and exult in jubilation over your goodness.

Abba Father, God of all goodness, add on everything this day to help me on my way to you, on my pilgrim way of faith to the eternal home.

You, God of healing, you know how much I want to become well again. I wish to do what is in my power to promote my healing. Ever so much from my heart do I beg you: Help me to stride forward on the way of healing.

Whatever this day brings me, for this already do I thank you, and in everything praise your Abba-Father Name.

And already do I greatly rejoice over that awakening which will gather me up wholly into the praising of your love.

Amen

DURING THE DAY

But let all who take refuge in you rejoice;
   let them ever sing for joy.

Psalm 5:11

Abba Father, dear Father in heaven! What happiness I experience when I consider the fact that, in union with your Son Jesus, I can name you our Abba Father, my Abba Father, with full confidence, and thereby know that the breath of the love which goes out from you and your Son prays and breathes in me.

So you are for me the Father in heaven; for a piece of heaven is actually in me when I pray Abba! Father in heaven!

Often have you encouraged me by pronouncing your name of Father. Illness then has not been able to disturb me so very much. Forevermore will I look to Jesus: for anyone who sees him sees you. He takes me now and with my final intake of breath right into his breath of love, which lets him say in prayer: "Abba Father! into your hands I place my breath, my spirit!" In union with him I entrust myself wholly to your love.

And then when the day of my life is running short, I will, with the last inbreathing, say "Abba Father," and with my earthly life breathing out, leave it into your loving hands.

Amen

IN THE EVENING

O Lord, our Sovereign,
>how majestic is your name in all the earth!
You have set your glory above the heavens.

Psalm 8:1

Yes, ineffable is thy glorious name, thou the All Highest. Still more glorious is that name of yours which you revealed to Moses: the *I-am-there*. Unsurpassable is the definitive revelation in Jesus, the Immanuel, *God-is-with-us* who has enabled us to name you Abba Father, in union with him and in the strength of the eternal Breath. Even this very day you have let me experience ever and again that you are the *I-am-there*, the *God-is-with-us*.

Your only begotten Son who has named himself Son of Adam, Son of Man, was exultant with joy because he was at liberty to tell us your name, the name of Father. And he rejoiced even in the holy Breath because it was through him that you revealed all that to us, men and women of no account.

On the evening of this day and with an eye on the evening of life to which I am drawing near, I wish to honor your name of Father with a great big trustfulness. You know, better than I do, what is harmful to me, and what is beneficial. You take care of me, immeasurably better than doctors and nurses provide for me.

Take from me everything that hinders me on the way to You and grant me everything that furthers my progress on this way!

Amen

IN THE NIGHT

[F]or you have been my help,
and in the shadow of your wings
I sing for joy
My soul clings to you;
your right hand upholds me.

Psalm 63:7-8

Father, dearest Father! When indeed the pious psalmist finds such unwavering refuge in you even before the coming of your Son into the universe, how much greater confidence should we have in your loving and fatherly care now that we know that you sent your only Son himself to die for our sins. What boundless trust should we now have as a result of this unearned gift!

Let me spend the whole night with Jesus in prayer in the delight of your love. Permit me to pray in your name, O Father, for the grace of your safety and the solace of your refuge.

As your humble follower, let me pray to you, the Lord of the heavens and the earth, using the holy and joyous breath of your love; let me never fail to thank you for the fatherly sacrifice of your Son.

Just as did your Son when he was at the point of death on the Mount of Olives and on the cross, let me murmur your Father-Name unceasingly in order to gain the strength and comfort that comes with being in the safe hands of your custody.

Following in your Son's trustful way, I will place my confidence in your healing plan and in your loving intentions for me; show me the road and give me confidence in this my darkest of nights.

And my gracious Father, if I stammer and mumble in my sleepiness, support me with your Holy Breath so that my weakness will not dim my wish to approach and to learn from your presence in prayer. Give me the strength to pray ever more in tune with you, my solicitous and holy Father.

Amen